Home Safety Checklist Guide and Caregiver Resources for Medication Safety, Driving, and Wandering

Laura Town and Karen Hoffman

D0967476

Omega Press
Zionsville, IN 46077

ISBN-13: 978-0-9969832-6-6
ISBN-10: 0-9969832-6-0

Production Credits:
Authors: Laura Town and Karen Hoffman
Publisher: Omega Press
Photos: All images used under license from Shutterstock.com

Social media connections:
Laura Town
Twitter: @laurawtown
LinkedIn: https://www.linkedin.com/in/lauratown

Karen Hoffman
LinkedIn: https://www.linkedin.com/in/karen-hoffman-91502b62/

CONTENTS

HOME SAFETY CHECKLIST GUIDE AND CAREGIVER RESOURCES FOR MEDICATION SAFETY, DRIVING, AND WANDERING

One hallmark of Alzheimer's disease is a decrease in cognitive functioning (information processing or thinking). The individual with Alzheimer's disease has a hard time making rational decisions, recognizing familiar people and places, and performing activities that were once routine. Because of their slower information processing, individuals with Alzheimer's disease may find themselves in dangerous situations, such as wandering unfamiliar streets, driving with slowed reaction times, stumbling over obstacles, or using home appliances incorrectly. As a caregiver, you can incorporate many small changes into your loved one's home to help provide a safe environment.

As you make these changes, you will likely find that one painful aspect of caring for a loved one with Alzheimer's disease is trying to balance their psychological need for independence with their physical safety. Alzheimer's disease can progress slowly or quickly, so the need for safety modifications may be urgent or may be postponed. In my dad's case, he was a high-functioning individual, so he hid his symptoms for years before we realized what was happening. Once we did understand the extent of his cognitive disabilities, we had no other choice but to move him closer to us. The jarring effect of the move precipitated a rapid decline in cognitive ability, which made it all the more urgent to modify Dad's home and make it safe for him.

Some of the items on the checklists throughout this chapter will be applicable to your situation now, and some will be applicable in the future as your loved one progresses through the disease. Know that implementing some of these changes may cause conflict between you and your loved one. In addition, your loved one may be scared, confused, or angry because they do not understand why all the changes are necessary. Unfortunately, your loved one's decline will eventually reach a point where you simply cannot respect your loved one's wishes because it would place them in physical danger. Fighting with your loved one is the last thing that you want to do, but know in your heart that you are doing the best you can with an intolerable situation.

Home Safety

Assuming your loved one is no longer working, they will likely be spending most of their time at home. Therefore, their home should be a safe place where they have reduced chances of falling, getting burned or cut, locking themselves in or out, and ingesting hazardous materials.

Fall Prevention

Older adults, even those without significant cognitive impairment, are at high risk of falling, which may result in fractured bones or other injuries. Older adults with a fractured hip have a higher chance of complications, including death within one year of injury. Individuals with Alzheimer's disease are at an even higher risk of falling than other older adults, because they may not process the presence of obstacles, they have a reduced sense of balance, and they

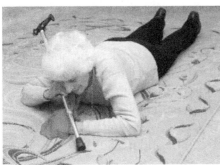

may make poor decisions about climbing and reaching. The thought of your loved one falling is likely one of the many nightmares you have as a caregiver. It was one that I had, even more so because my dad needed glasses to see and would refuse to wear them.

Credit: Stephen Rudolph

Preventing falls should be a high priority for you and your loved one. For me, the key to keeping Dad from falling was making sure that he had good, sturdy shoes on at all times (we used Velcro shoes as Dad would take out shoelaces and hide them) and keeping every room free of clutter. The checklists below provide some simple home changes you can make to help reduce the risk of falling.

Checklist: Emergency Alert system

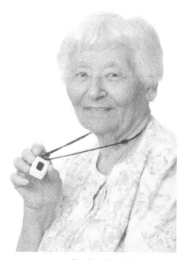

Credit: Paul Vasarhelyi

- ☐ Enroll your loved one in an emergency alert system such as Lifeline. With Lifeline and many other emergency alert systems, your loved one will wear a pendant with a button they can push to call for help if they fall. Lifeline now also has an auto-alert option that calls for help if it detects a fall and your loved one is unable to push the button.

- ☐ Extra emergency alert buttons can be mounted near the floor in common areas or in areas that an individual may land when they fall, such as the bottom of the stairway.

- ☐ You can order a Lifeline system online at https://www.lifeline.philips.com/ or call at 1-844-448-1403.

- ☐ Other emergency alert companies are listed in the Resources at the end of this book.

- ☐ Keep emergency contact numbers in easy reach of all phones. Program phones with speed dial for caregivers and emergency personnel, and make a list of the numbers in large font (e.g., 1 = daughter, 2 = police, etc.) and place it next to the phone. If desired, you could use photos to accompany the list. Leave clear, simple directions next to the phone for your loved one to follow.

Checklist: Outdoor modifications

- ☐ Keep walkways clear of debris.

- ☐ Fix loose or uneven steps.

- ☐ Add a railing next to walkways and stairs.

- ☐ Install a ramp to the front and back doors.

Checklist: Indoor modifications

Kitchen:

- ☐ Keep commonly-used dishes and utensils within easy reach to prevent climbing and reaching.

- ☐ If you need to polish the floor, use a nonslip cleaner. You may need to test several cleaners to determine which one works best for your flooring. Encourage your loved one to stay out of the kitchen when the floor is wet.

- ☐ Clean up spills immediately.

Bathroom:

- ☐ Remove all rugs that may slip; secure any remaining rugs or use nonskid mats. Rugs can be secured using nonslip rubber rug pads, double-sided tape, or glue. Different floor types will need different methods of securing a rug, and different rugs may need different methods as well, depending on the rug backing.

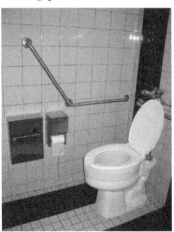

Credit: Carolyn Brule

- ☐ Add nonslip decals to the bottom of the shower or tub.

- ☐ Install a faucet cover in the bathtub to reduce injury if your loved one falls.

4

- ☐ Install grab bars in the shower and next to the toilet.

- ☐ Install a raised toilet seat.

- ☐ Install an anchored shower bench and a hand-held sprayer.

- ☐ Install a walk-in shower or tub to prevent having to climb over the side of the tub.

- ☐ Living spaces:

- ☐ Keep all walking areas free from clutter.

- ☐ Remove or secure rugs that may cause tripping.

- ☐ Make sure all electrical cords are secured to the floor and out of walking paths.

- ☐ Remove low furniture that may present a tripping hazard. Low furniture is furniture that is below knee-level, such as a coffee table.

- ☐ Encourage the use of assistive devices when walking; ensure that walking paths are wide enough to accommodate use of assistive devices.

- ☐ Provide your loved one with good, sturdy shoes that have rubber soles to prevent slipping. Make sure they wear the shoes at all times except when sleeping. Shoes with Velcro straps are preferred because some individuals with Alzheimer's disease may forget how to tie their shoes, leaving laces loose; or they may remove shoelaces, increasing the chances of the shoes falling off. This then presents another tripping hazard.

- ☐ Provide adequate lighting of all hallways and living spaces, especially at night. Use nightlights or motion-sensing lights as necessary. Because individuals with Alzheimer's disease have visual difficulties, inadequate lighting can cause confusion and misperceptions.

- ☐ Install handrails in all stairways; handrails should extend beyond the first and last steps.

- [ ] Install safety gates at the top and bottom of stairways. Be sure to install a gate that works best with your loved one's stairs and not one that tips easily.

- [ ] Add nonskid, colored strips to each stair. This helps define the stairs for individuals who have difficulty with depth perception due to similar colors.

- [ ] Be aware that pets can easily become tripping hazards, especially if they are a similar color as the carpet. If necessary, you may need to find these pets a new home.

Bedroom:

- [ ] Place clothing and shoes in easy-to-reach locations.

- [ ] Install side rails on the bed or use a hospital bed.

- [ ] Anticipate needs that might require your loved one to walk at night; make sure they have gone to the bathroom and are not hungry or thirsty before bedtime.

Hazard Safety

It is hard to understand how a diseased mind works. Individuals with Alzheimer's disease often have impaired perception and judgment. Therefore, they may not realize that something is dangerous. For example, they may touch a hot stove, eat a poisonous plant, or drink a clear liquid that happens to be bleach. They may not even understand the most basic activities, even if it's something that has been routine for them in the past. For example, my dad tried to make a frozen pizza, which he was an expert at, having been a bachelor for some time. One day he just turned on the burners and placed the cardboard box with the pizza on top. We are fortunate that he didn't burn himself or burn the house down. From that moment on, I made sure that his fridge was stocked with foods such as sandwiches, and we had Meals on Wheels bring him warm meals.

When caring for someone with Alzheimer's disease, you should learn to never underestimate a potential hazard. As a caregiver, removing hazardous substances or keeping them in a locked cabinet could save your loved one from potential injury or death. Hazard safety tips for individuals with Alzheimer's disease are included in the checklists below.

Checklist: Fire safety

- ☐ Make sure that smoke detectors are installed to code and working; change batteries at least once a year.

- ☐ Keep fire extinguishers in easily accessible locations; you should have one in every room if possible.

- ☐ Use child safety covers for all outlets when not in use.

- ☐ Keep matches and lighters locked up or out of reach.

- ☐ Consider disabling the stove, oven, and microwave when not in use. For example, remove the knobs of the stove and oven or install a hidden circuit breaker.

- ☐ If you decide to keep the microwave or stove functional, place clear, simple directions next to it for your loved one to follow. Make sure papers stay clear of the heating elements.

- ☐ If you decide to disable the microwave, stove, or oven, consider contacting Meals on Wheels to deliver hot meals to your loved one. Contact information is provided in the Resources at the end of this book.

- ☐ Remove space heaters and hot plates; do not let your loved one control settings for electric blankets or heating pads.

- ☐ Remove the fuel source for all grills when not in use.

- ☐ Supervise or restrict smoking. If your loved one must smoke, make sure someone is with them at all times. Cigarettes can be a fire hazard if left on flammable material.

- ☐ Supervise the use of the fireplace and candles; always extinguish the fire when leaving your loved one alone in a room with an open flame.

Checklist: Chemical safety

☐ Store household cleaning products and other chemicals in a locked cabinet.

☐ Keep all vitamins and medications in a locked cabinet.

☐ Clearly label all chemicals and medications.

☐ Keep alcohol in a locked cabinet. Monitor and discourage alcohol use, because alcohol can increase confusion.

☐ Keep poison control phone numbers in a convenient location. Information for the national poison control center is provided at in the Resources at the end of this book.

Checklist: Gun safety

☐ Remove firearms from the home; if this is not an option, lock the unloaded firearms in a gun safe to which your loved one does not have a key or combination.

☐ Lock bullets in a separate location from firearms. Bullets may present a choking hazard for individuals with Alzheimer's disease.

☐ Keep firearms unloaded when not in use.

Checklist: Personal safety

☐ Label or color code hot (red) and cold (blue) water faucets or install a faucet with only one handle that controls both hot and cold water.

☐ Set the hot water heater to 120 °F to avoid scalding. If your loved one's hot water heater temperature control is not reliable, consider replacing the hot water heater with a more reliable unit.

☐ Place red tape around heating sources to deter your loved one from touching it when hot.

☐ Remove or lock up sharp objects such as knives, razors, and scissors.

- ☐ Only allow your loved one to use an electric razor for shaving to prevent cuts.

- ☐ Consider disabling the garbage disposal, as individuals with Alzheimer's disease may stick their hand or other items into the disposal when it is running.

- ☐ Put away small appliances such as toasters and blenders when not in use.

- ☐ Use appliances that have an auto-shut-off feature.

- ☐ Keep appliances away from water sources, including bathroom appliances such as hair dryers and electric razors.

- ☐ Keep the refrigerator clear of spoiled foods, because your loved one may not be able to smell that the food is bad.

- ☐ Remove small items that may be easily swallowed; lock the "junk" drawer that may contain these items.

- ☐ Remove plastic fruit and magnets that may be mistaken for food and eaten.

- ☐ Replace breakable glass with plastic. This applies to glass tables, glass shower doors, drinking glasses, and ceramic plates.

- ☐ Mark windows and glass doors with decals to help your loved one see the glass panes.

- ☐ Make sure that carbon monoxide detectors are installed and working properly; change batteries at least once a year. Carbon monoxide detectors should be placed near sleeping areas and main living areas but not close to a furnace unit.

- ☐ Remove fish tanks or keep them out of reach, because they pose an electrocution hazard.

- ☐ Remove poisonous plants from the home.

- ☐ Store power tools in a locked space to which your loved one does not have a key.

- ☐ Disable automatic locks so your loved one does not get locked out accidentally.

- ☐ Hide an extra set of house keys outside in case your loved one locks everyone out.

- ☐ Install coverings or doors to hide rooms that may pose a hazard to your loved one.

- ☐ Have a first aid kit readily available.

- ☐ Keep emergency contact numbers in easy reach of all phones.

Medication Safety

Older adults, including individuals with Alzheimer's disease, often take a variety of medications for chronic diseases or conditions. Because of their deteriorating memory, individuals with Alzheimer's disease may forget to take their medication or may take the wrong

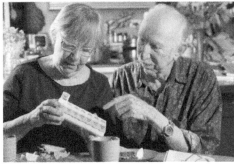

dose. As a caregiver, one of your responsibilities will be to make sure your loved one takes the appropriate medications at the right doses on the schedule prescribed by the physician. Safety precautions related to medications are listed below.

Credit: CREATISTA

Checklist: Medication safety

- ☐ Keep a complete and detailed list of your loved one's prescription medications, over-the-counter medications, vitamins, and herbal supplements with you at all times, including name, purpose, dose, and schedule.

- ☐ Discuss potential side effects and drug interactions with each healthcare provider.

- ☐ Keep a list of your loved one's drug allergies with you to discuss when receiving new medications.

- ☐ Supervise your loved one when they take medications to ensure that the correct medication is taken at the correct time; this will help prevent overdosing or under-dosing.

- ☐ If your loved one has a complex medication schedule, consider hiring a home health aide for one hour per day to make sure the medicine is taken appropriately.

- ☐ If your loved one has difficulty swallowing, ask the physician if there are other formulations of the medication your loved one can take, such as a liquid form. If you need to crush a pill, speak with the physician or pharmacist first, because some medications may become harmful or ineffective when crushed.

- ☐ If a physician has stated that medications can be mixed with food, mix medications with soft foods such as applesauce or ice cream.

- ☐ Use a pill box organizer to plan your loved one's medication schedule.

- ☐ Develop a routine for giving medication to your loved one.

- ☐ Always provide clear, simple, and step-by-step instructions to your loved one when taking medications.

- ☐ If your loved one refuses to take the medication, don't force them. Stop and try again later.

Staying Home Alone

Many individuals with Alzheimer's disease, especially if they are in the advanced stages of disease, should not be left at home alone. As a caregiver, how do you know when it is no longer safe for your loved one to be home alone? The questions in the checklist below are a good way to gauge the safety of leaving your loved one at home alone.

Checklist: *Is it safe to leave your loved one at home alone?*

- ☐ Is your loved one able to walk independently?

- ☐ Can your loved one safely get up and down from chairs, the bed, or the toilet?

- ☐ Can your loved one safely shower without supervision?

- ☐ Can your loved one get dressed by himself or herself?

- ☐ Does your loved one have any swallowing or eating difficulties?

- ☐ Does your loved one know the difference between safe and harmful items to eat or drink?

- ☐ Is your loved one able to safely take their prescribed medications?

- ☐ Does your loved one try to pursue hobbies that may no longer be safe, such as woodworking, cooking, or smoking?

- ☐ Is your loved one able to safely use the stove, oven, and microwave?

- ☐ Can your loved one safely use indoor and outdoor appliances and tools?

- ☐ Is your loved one prone to wandering?

- ☐ Does your loved one tend to get lost or disoriented in familiar places?

- ☐ If your loved one commonly uses public transportation to get around, can they get off at the right stops, and do they know how to ask for directions?

- ☐ Can your loved one repeat their phone number and address to a stranger?

- ☐ Does your loved one demonstrate warning signs for suicide?

- [ ] Does your loved one easily become confused when under stress?

- [ ] Does your loved one recognize dangerous situations, such as fire?

- [ ] Does your loved one show signs of agitation, depression, or withdrawal when left alone for long periods of time?

- [ ] Can your loved one use the phone to call for help?

- [ ] Would your loved one know what to do in case of an emergency or disaster?

You should reevaluate your loved one's ability to stay home alone frequently as their disease progresses, because what is safe for your loved one today may not be safe tomorrow. If you feel comfortable leaving your loved one alone after answering the questions in the list above, a few additional safety measures may help keep your loved one safe while they are home alone.

Checklist: Safety measures for loved ones who live alone

- [ ] Enroll your loved one in an emergency alert program, such as the MedicAlert® + Safe Return® program. In this program, your loved one wears a MedicAlert® bracelet that identifies them as being memory impaired. If they wander outside the house or get separated from you in public, the person who finds your loved one can call the number on the bracelet. Your loved one's identification number is then matched with your caregiver information so that your loved one can be safely returned to you. There is an initial and annual renewal cost for this program, which is run by the Alzheimer's Association. Applicants can enroll at medicalert.org/safereturn or by calling 1-888-572-8566.

- [ ] Before you leave your loved one alone, reassure them that you will only be gone a short time.

- [ ] Remind your loved one to call you or another family member or friend if they need help.

- Place important phone numbers next to each phone with step-by-step instructions for calling.

- Provide distractions for your loved one while you are out, such as favorite movies or games.

- Ask another family member or friend to check on your loved one while you are away, with either a phone call or a visit.

- Post large notes around the house reminding your loved one where you are and when you will be back.

- Place signs on the doors to prevent wandering outside, such as "Stop" or "Do Not Leave."

If your loved one has reached a point where it is no longer safe for them to be home alone, you can use several strategies to provide a break for yourself or some time to run errands.

Checklist: Strategies for additional care for your loved one

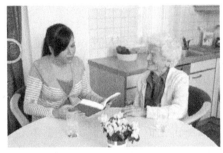

Credit: Lisa S.

- Ask a family member, friend, or neighbor to visit with your loved one while you are away.

- Invite a friend or family member to accompany you and your loved one on your errands.

- Hire a trusted individual to sit with your loved one while you are out.

- Hire a trained dementia professional or home health aide to care for your loved one.

- Place your loved one in an Adult Day Care Center while you are at work.

- ☐ Contact your local Meals on Wheels to deliver meals to your loved one.

- ☐ Consider placing your loved one in a full-time care facility.

- ☐ If a physician suggests that your loved one may be within six months of death, hiring hospice is a good option for additional care.

Wandering

Because dementia destroys brain cells responsible for memory and thinking, sixty percent of people with dementia will wander away from home at any time of the day or night or wander away from their loved ones when they are in public. Older adults with dementia who wander away from home often suffer serious injury or death if they are not found within the first 24 hours. Therefore, recognizing warning signs of wandering, preventing wandering, and being prepared in case your loved one wanders are all important tasks for caregivers.

Warning Signs for Wandering

As a caregiver, being able to recognize signs of wandering is an important first step for preventing wandering behavior. Wandering may be triggered by restlessness, anxiety, memory loss, disorientation, or physical needs such as hunger, thirst, or the urge to use the bathroom. Some warning signs are listed in the checklist below.

Checklist: Warning signs for wandering

- ☐ Coming back from a drive or walk later than usual.

- ☐ Not being able to use keys or understand their purpose.

- ☐ Wanting to go home, even when they are at home.

- ☐ Having a hard time remembering their name or address.

- ☐ Getting off at the wrong stop when taking public transportation.

- ☐ Trying to go to work even though they are no longer working.

- ☐ Talking about going to a favorite location from the past that is not near their home.

- ☐ Asking where current or past family and friends are.

- ☐ Searching for a person or item that was lost at one time in the past.

- ☐ Restlessness and excessive pacing.

- ☐ Acting nervous in public or crowded areas.

- ☐ Appearing lost in a new or changed environment.

- ☐ Appearing more confused in the early evenings (known as "sundowning").

- ☐ Becoming lost or disoriented easily, even in familiar surroundings.

- ☐ Appearing to be participating in a productive activity without actually getting anything done.

- ☐ Trying to escape from a perceived threat, such as a strange visitor. Note that in the later stages of disease, even people they've known for many years may seem like strangers. In extreme cases, your loved one may even react violently to the perceived "intruder."

Preparing for Wandering

The likelihood of your loved one having at least one wandering episode is very high, even if you take every precaution to prevent wandering. Before this occurs, you should take several steps to be prepared for a wandering episode.

Checklist: Wandering preparations

- ☐ Enroll your loved one in an emergency response program such as MedicAlert® + Safe Return® and ensure that your loved one wears the alert bracelet at all times.

- [ ] Consider investing in a GPS tracking system for your loved one.

- [ ] Place an identification card and explanation of your loved one's condition in a purse or wallet that they are likely to take with them when they wander.

- [ ] If your loved one frequently takes public transportation, provide them with a map that shows their common stops, including their home stop. Even if your loved one won't use the map, others who stop to help will find it useful.

- [ ] Place ID labels in the individual's clothing.

- [ ] Have several recent photos and a description of your loved one available.

- [ ] Keep a piece of your loved one's worn, unwashed clothing in a plastic bag to aid in canine searches. Replace the clothing item every month to keep the scent strong, and wear gloves when handling the clothing to prevent contaminating the item with your scent.

- [ ] Notify the police and other emergency personnel in your area that your loved one has Alzheimer's disease and may wander. Provide them with a description of your loved one and other important information, such as name, home address, your contact information, medication, health conditions, and allergies.

- [ ] Notify neighbors of your loved one's condition and ask them to contact you if they ever see your loved one wandering alone.

- [ ] Make a list of people that you can call for help.

- [ ] Obtain the contact information for your state's Silver Alert program.

Wandering Prevention

My father wandered. Sometimes he would end up at a neighbor's house, peeking in their windows and scaring them. Other times, he ended up at local businesses. One owner of a Subway sandwich shop was kind enough to recognize Dad, drive him home, and call me. Other wandering cases do not turn out so well. Alzheimer's patients can end up wandering and getting hurt by cars or end up in the cold, freezing. Once your loved one starts wandering, you must have a plan in place for 24-hour care. Once Dad started wandering, we hired 24-hour home health aides to sit with him. Any 24-hour solution to wandering will be expensive, but you likely will not have a choice.

Preventing episodes of wandering should begin long before your loved one begins wandering. Keep in mind that your loved one may not only wander from home. They may also wander away from you in public places. Preventing wandering episodes is especially important in extreme weather, such as extreme cold in winter, extreme heat in summer, or during storms. In addition to the preparedness steps above, practical steps to prevent wandering episodes are included in the checklist below.

Checklist: Wandering prevention tips

- ☐ Do not leave your loved one unsupervised in an unfamiliar location or alone at home.

- ☐ Make sure your loved one gets enough exercise; physical activity is as important for individuals with Alzheimer's disease as it is for any other older adult.

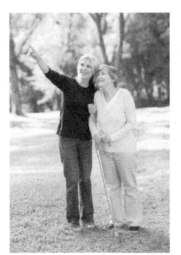

- ☐ Keep a regular schedule of supervised daily activities such as folding laundry, sweeping, and preparing dinner.

- ☐ Provide special, meaningful activities for your loved one to participate in during the day, such as visiting with friends or going for a walk.

Credit: michaeljung

- Provide a room free of clutter in which your loved one can safely pace.

- If your loved one appears restless, make sure all their basic needs are met, especially eating, drinking, and toileting. If their basic needs are met, engage them in physical activity such as going for a walk together or engage them in a favorite TV program or other activity. Reassure them and make them feel loved and appreciated.

- Monitor your loved one's wandering patterns, especially any behaviors or events that may indicate that wandering is likely to happen soon. When you identify these behaviors, distract your loved one with an activity or take care of any needs that may be prompting wandering behaviors.

- Reassure your loved one if they feel lost, disoriented, or abandoned. Use simple phrases to encourage them to stay home, such as "you don't need to go in to work today" or "we decided to stay here tonight." Do not try to convince them that their reality is incorrect, because this will enhance their agitation.

- Identify bathrooms and other common rooms with large signs to help your disoriented loved one find their way.

- Place locks high and low on the door, and install locks with different opening mechanisms. This keeps the locks out of the direct line of sight and increases the difficulty of opening the door.

- Camouflage doors by painting them the same color as the wall or covering them with a window hanging or cloth.

- Cover door knobs with a cloth the same color as the door or install child safety knob covers.

- Place "STOP," "CLOSED," or "DO NOT ENTER" signs on external doors.

- Install buzzers or alarms that sound when an outside door is opened. Make sure these are loud enough for you to hear when you are sleeping.

- ☐ Install safety locks on windows.

- ☐ Install motion detectors that will alert you when your loved one is moving around, especially at night.

- ☐ If your loved one tends to wander at night, make sure that important items such as a glass of water, eyeglasses, clock, source of light, tissues, and telephone are next to them by the bed.

- ☐ Keep coats, shoes, keys, hats, purses, and wallets out of sight, because many older individuals will not leave home without these items.

- ☐ Fence in your yard with a high wooden fence that does not have footholds for climbing. Use locked gates to prevent easy access.

- ☐ Cover swimming pools and restrict access so your loved one does not become injured or drown.

- ☐ Control access to house keys, car keys, and cash to eliminate nonwalking methods of wandering (cars, buses, etc.).

- ☐ Avoid busy places that may cause confusion, such as shopping malls.

- ☐ Consult with a physician to determine if medication can help reduce wandering or if any of your loved one's medications may induce wandering.

What to Do if Your Loved One Has Wandered

You have done everything in the above lists, yet your loved one has wandered away from home unattended and you don't know where to find them. What should you do now? Following the step-by-step instructions below will help you find your loved one as quickly as possible.

Checklist: Steps for searching for your loved one

- ☐ Search the immediate area for no more than 15 minutes. Check nearby businesses or parks that your loved one may visit frequently.

- ☐ If a quick search does not locate your loved one, call 911 or your local equivalent immediately.

- ☐ Call your list of friends, family, and neighbors who have offered to help you search for your loved one.

- ☐ Distribute information to the search party, including a photo and current information such as clothing, height, and weight. If the police have search dogs, provide them with a piece of your loved one's scented clothing.

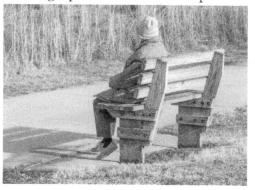

- ☐ Pinpoint areas of danger and search there first. These areas may include bodies of water, dense foliage, steep terrain, bus stops, busy highways, or tunnels.

Credit: Leigh Trail

- ☐ Search in the direction of your loved one's dominant hand (i.e., are they right-handed or left-handed?). People tend to turn first in that direction.

- ☐ Search areas that may be familiar to your loved one, such as a park, old work location, former home, church, or favorite store.

- ☐ If a thorough search of the surrounding area does not find your loved one, call your state's Silver Alert program.

Driving

Impaired judgment, slowed reaction times, and impaired vision interpretation combine to make driving dangerous for individuals with Alzheimer's disease. However, a diagnosis of Alzheimer's disease does not automatically mean that your loved one can no longer drive safely. As a caregiver, you will need to observe your loved one's driving patterns to help discern when your loved one needs to give up driving, because all individuals with Alzheimer's disease will eventually reach a point when they no longer have the judgment and memory needed to drive safely. Restricting or banning your loved one's driving privileges may result in tension and defiance, because they interpret it as taking away their independence. However, for the safety of your loved one and others on the road, you must stand firm when it is time to take the keys away.

Taking my dad's keys away was one of the top five worst days of my life. I hated doing something that was so hurtful to him and signified the end of his independence. I also knew that his inability to drive would increase my caregiving burden. He was mad at me for days and wouldn't speak to me. Our relationship became so acrimonious that I ended up telling him that if he passed the driving test at the Department of Motor Vehicles that I would give him his keys back. I then printed off a practice written test and gave it to him. He returned it to me with only one question answered, and we never spoke of his driving again. I also moved the car into storage so he could no longer see it out his window. These strategies helped ease this painful transition.

The loss of driving abilities is inevitable for individuals with Alzheimer's disease. But when do you know when your loved one has gotten to the point of no longer being able to drive safely? The questions below can help you decide when it is appropriate to tell your loved one that they can no longer drive.

Checklist: Is it safe for my loved one to be driving?

- ☐ Does your loved one understand the purpose of keys?

- ☐ Does your loved one understand the difference between drive, reverse, and park?

- ☐ Can your loved one remember how to get to familiar places?

- ☐ Does your loved one forget where they are going during the trip?

- ☐ Can your loved one repeat their name, address, and phone number to a stranger when they are lost?

- ☐ Is your loved one slow to make decisions when driving?

- ☐ Is your loved one able to anticipate dangerous situations?

- ☐ Does your loved one have a shortened attention span?

- ☐ Is your loved one easily distracted while driving?

- ☐ Does your loved one become confused or angry while driving?

- ☐ Does your loved one become drowsy while driving?

- ☐ Does your loved one consistently obey traffic laws and signals?

- ☐ Has your loved one had a recent increase in accidents or traffic violations?

- ☐ Have you noticed any new dents or scratches on the car?

- ☐ Does your loved one drive at inappropriate speeds?

- ☐ Does your loved one appropriately use the gas and brake pedals?

- ☐ Does your loved one make spatial errors when driving, such as hitting the curb or wandering between lanes?

- ☐ Does your loved one have trouble negotiating turns, especially left-hand turns?

- ☐ Is your loved one able to park correctly?

- ☐ Do you feel safe riding in the car when your loved one is driving? Would you feel safe having your children ride with your loved one?

Once you have decided that you need to prevent your loved one from driving, how should you go about it? The discussion must be handled with care to avoid alienating or agitating your loved one. Consider some of the tips below when you are faced with this difficult discussion.

Checklist: Tips for discussing driving limitations

- ☐ Have the discussion about driving long before your loved one is no longer able to drive to prepare them for this inevitable outcome. Involving your loved one in the decision process will help the transition go more smoothly.

- ☐ Recognize that you may need to have this discussion multiple times. For the person with Alzheimer's disease, it is better to have several short conversations than one long conversation.

- ☐ Discussions should be timed with other changes, such as changes in medication that may affect driving.

- ☐ Remember that a single instance of poor driving doesn't mean that your loved one should stop driving. However, it does mean that your loved one should be monitored regularly for poor driving patterns.

- ☐ Document unsafe driving behaviors, and use them as evidence for why your loved one should no longer be driving.

- ☐ Avoid overreacting to driving incidences. Save the conversation about driving safety until after the immediate problem is resolved.

- ☐ Provide a simple explanation for why your loved one cannot drive. Focus on the disease rather than the individual as the reason to stop driving. Because thinking is slower for individuals with Alzheimer's disease, you may need to repeat the same simple sentence multiple times before they understand.

- ☐ Encourage your loved one to stop driving voluntarily. Appeal to your loved one's sense of responsibility to not endanger others on the road.

- ☐ Provide advantages of no longer driving, such as saving money on gas, insurance, and car repairs.

- Acknowledge your loved one's feelings about losing the capability to drive; confirm your unconditional love and support. Be patient but firm in your decision.

- Ask your loved one's physician to issue a "do not drive" prescription. Use the prescription to reinforce that they can no longer drive. Your loved one may take the news better coming from a doctor than from you or another friend or family member.

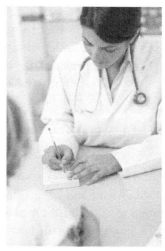

Credit: wavebreakmedia

- Have your loved one take a driving test administered by the Department of Motor Vehicles. They should be tested at least annually until they are no longer able to drive.

Although your loved one can no longer drive themselves independently, they will still need to be transported to doctor's appointments, activities, and errands. Some solutions for making sure your loved one still has ready transportation are listed below.

Checklist: Alternative driving options

- Slowly transition driving responsibilities to others. Alternative sources of transportation that are safe for your loved one can include family members or friends, a taxi service, or a special transportation service for older adults. Assisted living facilities also often provide group transportation services.

- Find ways to reduce your loved one's need to drive, such as having groceries and medications delivered.

- Tell your loved one that you are driving as a treat for them so they can sit back and enjoy the ride.

- When possible, walk with your loved one to your destination, and make it a special occasion.

- Even if your loved one is no longer able to drive, they may be able to walk to neighboring businesses on their own to retain some independence. However, only allow them to walk in safe places that have sidewalks and slow traffic, and do not allow them to walk alone if they have a pattern of wandering or getting lost.

- When you are driving your loved one on errands, do not leave your loved one alone in a parked car.

If your loved one insists that they can still drive safely even though you and others have documented that they cannot, you may need to take drastic measures as a last resort to prevent your loved one from driving and endangering themselves and others. Some options for preventing your loved one from driving are included in the checklist below.

Checklist: Driving prevention tips

- Control access to the car keys. If your loved one insists on carrying keys, provide them with old keys that do not work.

- Disable the car by removing the distributor cap or battery, or have a mechanic install a "kill switch" that must be flipped before the car will start.

- Keep the car out of sight or at a different location. This will help your loved one not think about driving as much.

- If you do not need the vehicle, consider selling your loved one's car and using the money to pay for other modes of transportation.

Going Out

As a caregiver, you will often be responsible for your loved one when they need to leave the house. Most trips will be to familiar locations such as the doctor's office, grocery store, or church. However, your ability to take your loved one out will change as the disease progresses, and it's hard to know how they will react. For a period of time, for example, I was able to take my dad out to lunch on a daily basis. At one point, after lunch I would take Dad back to his assisted living facility and he would become violent, which was completely uncharacteristic of him. I talked to his geriatric psychologist and he told me that the abrupt change in surroundings could be triggering the episodes, so I was unable to take him to lunch again. In fact, he wasn't able to leave the facility again.

In addition to leaving the home for a short time, some occasions require your loved one to travel or be away from home for an extended period of time. These situations require extra effort and preparation.

Special Occasions

Your loved one may be invited to special occasions such as holiday parties, family gatherings, graduations, or birthday parties. These events will likely be in an unfamiliar, loud, and crowded location. All of these qualities can increase stress, agitation, and confusion for your loved one. Ways to help your loved one adapt to this new or changed environment are listed below.

Checklist: Participating in special occasions

- ☐ Prepare people coming to the party about changes in your loved one's condition so the visitors don't get too emotional and upset your loved one. Ask them not to discuss your loved one's disease or health with the individual who has Alzheimer's disease, because this also may upset them.

- ☐ Prepare a place where your loved one can go to escape the noise and stimulation. Your loved one may need to rest or just be alone for a few minutes to help decrease confusion, anxiety, and exhaustion.

- ☐ Be prepared for your loved one to think they are attending a special occasion in the past. Encourage your loved one to talk about the past event. Do not try to correct or reorient them, because this may cause more confusion and anxiety.

- ☐ If your loved one is unable to participate in the entire event, choose to attend the portion of the event that is most meaningful to your loved one.

- If your loved one is unable to attend the event, consider bringing the event to your loved one. For example, if your loved one cannot attend a wedding, a visit from the bride and groom may provide a special blessing to your loved one.

- Consider having the celebration at your loved one's home with just a small group of people. Multiple smaller parties will be easier for your loved one than one large party. Plan the party for your loved one's best time of day.

- If you will be hosting a large party, prepare your loved one ahead of time by discussing your plans. Use simple sentences, and remind them frequently.

- Involve your loved one in the planning and preparations. Even if they can't contribute as much as they once did, they will enjoy being involved and feeling needed.

- If visitors will be staying in the loved one's home, make sure they are aware of potential hazards such as leaving out medications or creating clutter that the loved one may trip over.

- When planning a party, stick to your favorite traditions rather than trying to do everything. For example, if the family's favorite tradition is frosting sugar cookies together, then make only frosted sugar cookies and not all the other Christmas treats you might normally have.

- Enlist help from others both in preparations and in caregiving during the event. Ask others to bring food for a potluck-style meal.

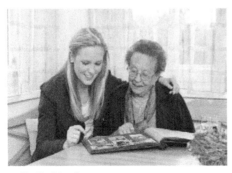

Credit: Lisa S.

- Plan quiet activities such as looking through a photo album rather than loud, boisterous activities such as playing games.

28

- [ ] If decorating for a holiday, choose a few subtle decorations that will not alter your loved one's environment too much. Too many changes may cause confusion because of changes to visual cues.

- [ ] Secure decorations so they do not fall or pose a tripping or fire hazard to your loved one. Be sure to monitor all flammable decorations at all times when your loved one is present.

Traveling

Some occasions, such as weddings or vacations, may require your loved one to travel by car or airplane. This will be another stressful situation for your loved one, especially if they have not flown or gone on long trips frequently in the past. The noise level, unfamiliar concourses, confined seating, and strange physical sensations will add to your loved one's confusion and stress level. Good tips to prepare for traveling are listed below.

Checklist: Traveling tips

- [ ] If possible, travel to known locations that are close to home. Plan to be away from home for only a few days.

- [ ] Travel during your loved one's best time of day, and choose the travel option that will cause the least anxiety for your loved one.

- [ ] Avoid traveling on peak travel days. It is also better to travel in the off-season when hotels and major activities will be less crowded.

- [ ] Avoid scheduling flights with tight connections, and try to fly direct if possible.

- [ ] Allow extra time for every step of the trip, from packing to arrival.

- [ ] Pack important documents such as medication information, travel itineraries, and contact information. Keep at least one copy with your loved one in case they wander and get lost.

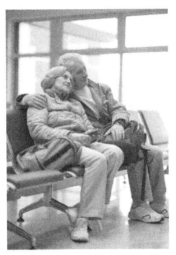

Credit: Ruslan Guzov

□ Pack activities, snacks, and water in a small bag for your loved one.

□ Never let your loved one travel unattended. It is not the job of the airline employees to make sure your loved one stays safe. Consider bringing someone along who can help with caregiving duties.

□ Get a letter from the doctor that states that your loved one has a cognitive impairment. This will help ease tensions with airport security if your loved one has trouble following directions.

□ Inform hotel and airline staff of your loved one's special needs before you arrive, and remind them of your loved one's needs when you arrive.

□ Consider requesting wheelchair support at your gate so that you have an airport employee to accompany you. Special considerations such as this often require at least 48 hours advance notice.

□ Use the restroom before getting on the plane to avoid having to use the on-board lavatory. If you think your loved one will need to use the bathroom on the plane, schedule the bathroom trip for about an hour before the end of the flight to avoid needing the bathroom when the seatbelt sign is turned on for landing.

□ Preboard the aircraft, and choose a middle or window seat for your loved one and an aisle seat for yourself so your loved one cannot wander without you noticing. If possible, sit on a side with only two seats.

- ☐ Request a hotel room designed for people with disabilities. Share a room with your loved one, and sleep in the bed nearest the door. Consider bringing along a travel door alarm to warn you if your loved one tries to leave the room.

- ☐ When you arrive at your hotel room or other accommodations, assess the room or house for hazards and remove them. If you are staying at someone's house, kindly ask them if you can remove the hazards for the duration of your stay.

- ☐ Stick to your loved one's normal schedule as much as possible. Keep meal and bed times the same, and bring along a favorite pillow or pair of pajamas.

- ☐ If you are enrolled in an emergency response program such as MedicAlert® + Safe Return®, alert the program that you will be traveling. Keep a recent photo of your loved one with you to show to people if they get lost.

- ☐ Find out contact information and directions to medical services at your destination.

- ☐ If your loved one is in an advanced stage of disease, suffers from incontinence, cannot perform most activities of daily living on their own, or gets confused easily, consider staying home.

Disaster Preparedness

If you live in an area that has frequent natural disasters, such as earthquakes, hurricanes, tornadoes, or forest fires, you need to have a plan in place to ensure the safety of your loved one with Alzheimer's disease. Your loved one may not be able to recognize or respond to danger, may wander outside and get lost, or may not know how to get

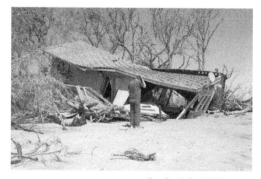

Credit: John Wollwerth

to a safe place before the disaster hits. Some ideas to help you and your loved one be prepared for a disaster are included in the checklist below.

Checklist: Disaster preparedness tips

- ☐ Put together an emergency kit in a waterproof container and store it in a convenient location. The kit should include items such as: copies of important documents and identification, extra medication and instructions, extra eyeglasses and hearing aid batteries, a recent picture of your loved one, basic first aid products, a flashlight with extra batteries, extra sets of clothing, incontinence products (if needed), bottled water, and favorite nonperishable food items. Different people have different needs, so consider your loved one's most basic needs and pack your emergency kit accordingly.

- ☐ Devise and practice an emergency exit plan. Make sure your emergency plan includes consideration of your loved one's specific needs, such as access to a walker or wheelchair. Update the plan frequently to reflect your loved one's changing capabilities.

- ☐ Assign one individual the responsibility of caring for your loved one during an emergency evacuation.

- ☐ When planning for a natural disaster or emergency, don't forget to include a plan for any pets your loved one has.

- ☐ Get to know your neighbors, and enlist them in helping you and your loved one during a natural disaster. Give your neighbors important information such as contact information of caregivers, family members, and medical services. Teach them about your loved one's habits and struggles, and teach them how to provide simple instructions to your loved one.

- ☐ If your loved one lives in a long-term care facility, learn about their emergency exit plan and find out who will be in charge of your loved one during the evacuation.

- ☐ Make sure your loved one always has an emergency alert bracelet on for identification.

- ☐ Write out a plan for who will care for your loved one if something happens to you.

- ☐ Make an inventory of your loved one's possessions, and make sure your loved one has adequate insurance coverage.

- ☐ Make your local law enforcement agency, fire department, emergency medical services, and hospitals aware of your loved one's condition. If an emergency occurs, they will know what to do if your loved one is confused.

- ☐ If you must go to a shelter or hotel for safety, make sure the staff knows about your loved one's condition.

- ☐ If you must evacuate to a hotel or shelter, use strategies to reduce your loved one's agitation such as taking a walk, talking calmly, or participating in an activity. Reassure your loved one that they are in the right place.

Elder Abuse

Individuals with Alzheimer's disease are often frustrating to work with because they do not understand, are forgetful, and may be prone to violence or defiance. These characteristics may cause caregivers to abuse the individual with Alzheimer's disease in order to get them to cooperate. Individuals with Alzheimer's disease are extremely susceptible to elder abuse because they often don't recognize that they are being abused, do not have the verbal or cognitive skills to report the abuse, and think that no one will believe their report of abuse because of their frequent confusion.

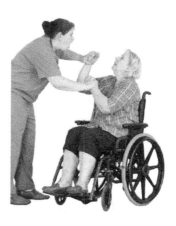

Credit: Sylvie Bouchard

Elder abuse can come in many different forms, as listed below, and it can occur as a single act or repeated acts. In most cases of repeated abuse, the abuser is someone the individual knows well, such as a close family member or friend. Elder abuse is also common in long-term care facilities, because caregivers often do not have the time or resources to handle the complex behaviors associated with Alzheimer's disease.

Checklist: Types of elder abuse

- ☐ **Physical abuse:** Physical injury because of beating, lashing, cutting, burning, or other physical assault.

- ☐ **Emotional abuse:** Emotional disturbance because of shouting, verbal insults, threats, harassment, or intimidation.

- ☐ **Sexual abuse:** Inappropriate touching that is forced on the individual or that they cannot consent to or understand; this can also include inappropriate sexual comments.

- ☐ **Financial abuse:** Withholding finances that will provide essential care for the individual; using the individual's finances in a way that is a disadvantage to the individual but an advantage to someone else; this is often a result of inappropriate use of a power of attorney or a result of strangers scamming an unsuspecting older adult with dementia.

- ☐ **Neglect:** Intentionally or unintentionally withholding food, water, shelter, medical care, hygiene care, and other basic necessities; this increases the individual's risk of physical or emotional harm.

- ☐ **Confinement:** Restraining or isolating the individual against their wishes.

- ☐ **Medical abuse:** Inappropriate prescription or withholding of anti-psychotics and other prescription drugs, restraints, catheters, and similar medical treatments.

Your loved one may be at risk for abuse both at home and at a care center. Caregivers, family members, and friends may abuse your loved one out of ignorance, frustration, or selfishness. How do you recognize if your loved one is being abused? You can look for some of the signs listed below.

Checklist: Signs of abuse

- ☐ Noticeable injuries such as bruises, broken bones, abrasions, or burns

- ☐ Matching bruises on the arms or throat may indicate rough grabbing

- ☐ Small round burn marks may indicate being touched with a burning cigarette

- ☐ Unexplained pain when moving

- ☐ Unexplained withdrawal from social activities

- ☐ Sudden changes in alertness or depression symptoms

- ☐ Bruises around the breast or genital areas

- ☐ Unexpected or unexplained withdrawals from a checking or savings account

- ☐ Increased occurrence of unpaid bills

- ☐ A new friend asks to help with the individual's banking

- ☐ Sudden changes to legal documents such as power of attorney or will

- ☐ Pressure ulcers

- ☐ Poor hygiene

- ☐ Unexpected weight loss

- ☐ Frequent arguments between your loved one and a specific person

Detecting abuse of an individual with Alzheimer's disease may be especially difficult because some of the signs of abuse, such as withdrawal or depression, are also common with disease progression even in the absence of abuse. Your consistent involvement in your loved one's life will allow you to more readily differentiate signs of abuse from signs of disease progression. As a caregiver and someone concerned about your loved one's physical and emotional safety, there are several ways you can help prevent or stop abuse, as stated in the checklist below.

Checklist: Ways to prevent elder abuse

- ☐ Be involved in your loved one's life.

- ☐ Undergo training in how to deal with the challenging behaviors that accompany Alzheimer's disease.

- ☐ Be aware of the care your loved one is receiving and the people your loved one interacts with daily; perform background or reference checks for people who will be caring for your loved one.

- ☐ Don't be afraid to ask questions of other caregivers and family members if you notice new injuries or behaviors.

- ☐ Ensure that your loved one's finances are being used for their best interests and not the interests of others.

- ☐ Be aware of individuals asking for money, including "salesmen" and other scammers. These individuals may use force or threats to con money out of your loved one.

- ☐ If you notice a caregiver that seems burned out or overburdened, offer to give them a break or refer them to a support group.

- ☐ If you suspect that your loved one is being abused, call national or state adult protective services or the police department. They will investigate your suspicions and bring charges against guilty parties if needed.

Keep in mind that because of your loved one's mental decline, you as a caregiver may also be susceptible to abuse by your loved one. Individuals with Alzheimer's disease may become aggressive and lash out at caregivers without provocation. No individual should have to live with the threat of abuse, even if it is coming from a loved one with dementia. If your loved one becomes abusive to you or other family members, seek help from medical professionals and loved ones.

Suicide

Many people who are diagnosed with Alzheimer's disease fear losing the ability to think, recognize their loved ones, and have meaningful interactions with the world around them. They also fear being a burden to their spouse, children, and friends based on their personal experiences with parents or others who had Alzheimer's disease. Therefore, many of them commit suicide or consider committing suicide before the disease progresses too far. In addition, there are many murder-suicide cases in which the healthy spouse kills their Alzheimer's-afflicted partner and then commits suicide. Some facts about suicide in patients with Alzheimer's disease or another form of dementia are listed below.

Checklist: Facts about Alzheimer's disease and suicide

☐ Individuals with a recent diagnosis of dementia are at higher risk for committing suicide, because they can still understand what the future may hold for them and their loved ones. The risk for suicide decreases as the disease progresses, because the individual loses the physical and mental capacity to commit suicide.

☐ Individuals with a history of depression and/or previous attempts to commit suicide are at higher risk of attempting suicide after a dementia diagnosis.

☐ Caucasians are more likely to commit suicide than other races, and men are more likely to commit suicide than women.

☐ A higher level of cognitive functioning is associated with an increased risk of suicide.

☐ The most common method of suicide is gunshot wound, which is why removing or locking guns is vitally important.

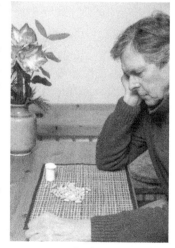

Credit: Miriam Doerr

37

- [ ] If firearms are unavailable, individuals with dementia may overdose on drugs, hang themselves, or jump from a height to commit suicide.

- [ ] Individuals in full-time care facilities are less likely to commit suicide, probably because of the increased monitoring and more advanced disease stage.

As a caregiver to your loved one with early stage Alzheimer's, how do you know if your loved one is contemplating suicide? Some warning signs are listed below.

Checklist: *Warning signs of suicide*

- [ ] Your loved one exhibits the classic signs of depression, including withdrawal, apathy, fatigue, irritability, sleep problems, and feelings of helplessness or hopelessness.

- [ ] Your loved one becomes more socially isolated than before their Alzheimer's diagnosis.

- [ ] Your loved one states that they would rather leave their money behind for their loved ones than spend it on a full-time care facility.

- [ ] Your loved one states that they would prefer death to being unable to care for themselves and being unable to recognize their loved ones.

- [ ] Your loved one discusses feeling like a burden. Many individuals will state that they intend to commit suicide before they decline as much as a parent or other loved one who suffered from Alzheimer's disease.

- [ ] Your loved one begins to plan what will happen after their death; they plan their funeral and start to give away prized possessions.

- [ ] Your loved one mentions that they are planning to commit suicide before they reach the advanced stages of the disease.

- [ ] Your loved one admits to having a plan for how they will commit suicide.

□ Your loved one wants to discuss the right time for them to take their own life. Most individuals plan to live as long as possible but commit suicide before the dementia becomes too severe.

If your loved one shows any of the above signs, what should you do? There are many potential options when caring for a loved one with Alzheimer's disease who is threatening to commit suicide. A few options are listed below.

Checklist: Responding to a suicidal loved one

□ Assess your loved one's situation. Do they live alone? Do they have a history of suicide?

□ Evaluate your loved one's ability to carry out their plan for suicide. Do they have both the physical and mental capacity to kill themselves? Do they have access to drugs or a firearm?

□ Consult with other family members about your loved one's condition and plan a strategy as a team.

□ Talk to your loved one about their suicidal thoughts. Affirm your loved one's feelings without implying that you want them to commit suicide.

□ Develop a safety plan with your loved one. This will encourage your loved one to call you or a trusted friend or family member before harming themselves.

□ Talk to a physician about your loved one's suicidal ideations. The physician may be able to prescribe a medication or suggest a counselor for your loved one.

□ Decrease your loved one's time alone. If your loved one lives alone at home, increase the number of times someone checks on them throughout the day. If your loved one lives in a full-time care facility, notify the staff and suggest frequent checks on your loved one.

Conclusion

Providing a safe environment for your loved one with Alzheimer's disease is a big task. New hazards may appear each day, and it can be exhausting keeping up with all the changes that are needed to keep your loved one safe. Know that whether you are doing something simple such as removing clutter or doing something drastic such as taking away their right to drive, you are acting in a way that protects your loved one from self-harm as well as from others who may harm them.

About the Authors

Laura Town

Laura Town has authored numerous publications of special interest to the aging population. She has expertise in the field of finance as a co-author on *Finance: Foundations of Financial Institutions and Management* published by John Wiley and Sons, and she has contributed to several online nursing courses and texts. She has also written for the American Medical Writers Association, and her 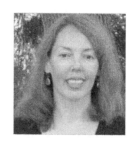 work has been published by the American Society of Journalists and Authors. As an editor, Laura has worked with Pearson Education, Prentice Hall, McGraw-Hill Higher Education, John Wiley and Sons, and the University of Pennsylvania to create both on-ground and online courses and texts. She is the former President of the Indiana chapter of the American Medical Writers Association.

Karen Hoffman

Karen (Kassel) Hoffman received her Ph.D. in pharmacology from the Department of Pharmacology and Experimental Neurosciences at the University of Nebraska Medical Center in Omaha, where she was the recipient of an American Heart Association fellowship and several regional and national awards for her research on G protein-coupled receptor signaling 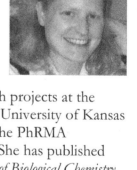 in airways. She then pursued post-doctoral research projects at the University of North Carolina–Chapel Hill and the University of Kansas Medical Center, again receiving fellowships from the PhRMA Foundation and the American Heart Association. She has published research in the *American Journal of Pathology*, *Journal of Biological Chemistry*, and *Journal of Pharmacology and Experimental Therapeutics*. In 2012, Karen joined the editorial staff at WilliamsTown Communications, an editing firm that specializes in educational products for undergraduate- and graduate-level students. At WTC, Karen specializes in producing educational products related to the sciences and healthcare. In addition, Karen is board-certified for editing life sciences (BELS-certified).

A Note from the Authors

Thank you for purchasing our book! Worldwide, over forty million people suffer from Alzheimer's disease, and that number is expected to increase significantly within the next fifteen years. In the United States, over five million people have the disease, and that is expected to triple by the year 2050.

Despite these large numbers, you may feel alone. I (Laura) know that when I started caring for my father, who had early-onset Alzheimer's disease, I felt alone. What helped was knowing that there are people, resources, and organizations that can help.

We recognize that caregivers have emotional, physical, and financial challenges. We hope that the information in the Alzheimer's Roadmap series will ease some of your stress. The steps included in this book can help you prepare for Alzheimer's disease or another terminal illness. All of the steps may not apply to every situation, but they will stimulate your thinking and get you moving forward in preparing for your future. In addition, we have included resources at the end of each book to provide additional information to help you through this process.

If you have any questions for us, feel free to post them on Laura Town's Amazon Author Central page or reach out via twitter: @laurawtown. We would appreciate it if you would take the time to review our book on Amazon, as our book's visibility on Amazon depends on reviews.

More Titles from Omega Press

Dementia, Alzheimer's Disease Stages, Treatments, and Other Medical Considerations

Advance Directives, Durable Power of Attorney, Wills, and Other Legal Considerations

Paying for Healthcare and Other Financial Considerations

Home Safety Checklist Guide and Caregiver Resources for Medication Safety,

Driving, and Wandering

Home Care, Long-term Care, Memory Care Units, and Other Living Arrangements

Enhancing the Activities of Daily Living

Nutrition for Brain Health: Fighting Dementia

Caregiver Resources: From Independence to a Memory Care Unit

Resources

Emergency Alert Systems

Philips Lifeline

Phone: 855-214-1363

Website: https://www.lifeline.philips.com/

Medic Alert + Alzheimer's Association Safe Return

2323 Colorado Blvd.

Turlock, CA 95380

Phone: 888-572-8566

Fax: 800-863-3429

Website: medicalert.org/safereturn

Silver Alert

Each state has its own program, so you will need to look up your state's information. However, the California Highway Patrol and the Texas Department of Public Safety offer comprehensive explanations of the program on their websites (https://www.chp.ca.gov/news-alerts/silver-alert and https://www.dps.texas.gov/dem/Operations/Alerts/SilverAlertOverview.htm). Note that the criteria listed on these websites may vary in your state.

Other emergency alert companies:

Alert1

Bay Alarm Medical

Care Innovations Link

Life Alert

LifeFone

LifeStation

Medical Guardian

MobileHelp

Rescue Alert

Website comparing companies: http://medical-alert-systems-review.toptenreviews.com/

Other

American Association of Poison Control Centers

515 Kind St., Suite 510

Alexandria, VA 22314

Phone: 800-222-1222

Email: info@aapcc.org

Website: http://www.aapcc.org

This website also contains a place to search for your local poison control center.

Meals on Wheels America

413 N. Lee St.

Alexandria, VA 22314

Phone: 888-998-6325

Fax: 703-548-5274

Email: info@mealsonwheelsamerica.org

Website: http://www.mealsonwheelsamerica.org

This website also contains a place to search for your local Meals on Wheels program.

Other books in the Alzheimer's Roadmap series

Dementia, Alzheimer's Disease Stages, Treatments, and Other Medical Considerations

Advance Directives, Durable Power of Attorney, Wills, and Other Legal Considerations

Paying for Healthcare and Other Financial Considerations

Home Safety Checklist Guide and Caregiver Resources for Medication Safety, Driving, and Wandering

Home Care, Long-term Care, Memory Care Units, and Other Living Arrangements

Enhancing the Activities of Daily Living

Nutrition for Brain Health: Fighting Dementia

Caregiver Resources: From Independence to a Memory Care Unit

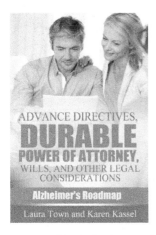

A preparatory guide to the legal documents, insurance, and other necessities for living with dementia

Advance Directives, Durable Power of Attorney, Wills, and Other Legal Considerations provides answers to the following questions and more:

- **How do I get a handle on my finances?** Find out what you need to do to gather information in order to prepare to pass on your financial information and assets, and early considerations for the task of passing on this wealth to others.
- **How do I transfer wealth to my loved ones?** You get a plan for the process of transferring wealth before or after death and a road map both for setting up joint ownership of accounts and preparing for the tax implications of wealth transfer.
- **What types of insurance should I have?** You get a walkthrough of the various types of insurance policies you'll need to consider, including long-term care insurance, disability insurance, and the different types of life insurance policy.
- **How do I know I've found a good insurance policy?** Checklists tell you things to watch out for as you choose a policy as well as outline the characteristics of good policies.
- **What legal documents for finances and healthcare do I need?** This book takes you through the ins and outs of creating durable powers of attorney for finances and healthcare, a last will and testament, a living trust, a living will, and advance directives.
- **Is there an electronic version of this book?** Yes, and it's free! You can find it at: **https://www.amazon.com/dp/B00OKD42TS**
- **Is there an audio version of this book?** Yes, there is. You can find it at: **https://adbl.co/2tQqMQF**

Living arrangements to preserve the dignity, independence, and safety of older adults with changing health needs

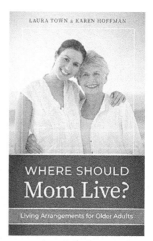

Where Should Mom Live? Living Arrangements for Older Adults provides answers to the following questions and more:

- **What are simple things I can do to help my loved one stay independent?** Learn simple things you can do to make your loved one's activities of daily living easier to accomplish on their own.
- **How can I keep my loved one living alone safe?** A range of home modifications can make your loved one's home a safer and more livable environment, some as simple and cost free as reducing clutter, removing tripping hazards, and increasing the space between pieces of furniture.
- **What if my loved one needs help living at home?** Understand the roles that home services, such as homemaker, companion, personal care, and home healthcare services, can play in helping your loved one live at home comfortably and securely.
- **What happens when my loved one needs to leave home?** From moving in with a caregiver to assisted living, full-time care facilities, memory care units, and psychiatric facilities, this book helps you navigate and choose the best options for your loved one while avoiding caregiver burnout and spotting signs to protect your loved one from elder abuse and exploitation.
- **Is there an electronic version of this book?** Yes, and it's free! You can find it at: **https://www.amazon.com/dp/B07F76PBB7**
- **Is there an audio version of this book?** Yes, there is. You can find it at: **https://adbl.co/2GYkhUE**

A guide to Alzheimer's disease progression and treatment

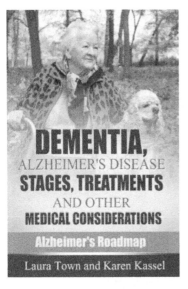

Dementia, Alzheimer's Disease Stages, Treatments, and Other Medical Considerations provides answers to the following questions and more:

- **What is Alzheimer's disease?** This book describes what Alzheimer's disease is, including its characteristics, warning signs, and risk factors.
- **What can my loved one with Alzheimer's disease expect?** Read detailed descriptions of the general stages of Alzheimer's disease, including what patients and caregivers can expect to see at each stage as the disease progresses.
- **What treatments are available?** A survey of prescription medications introduces you to the treatments available to help patients with Alzheimer's disease cope with the progression of the disease. Also find out which drugs to *avoid*.
- **What about clinical trials?** Clinical trials are important to finding a cure for Alzheimer's disease, but this book describes the precautions your loved one to consider before choosing to participate in them.
- **Is there an electronic version of this book?** Yes, and it's free! You can find it at: **https://www.amazon.com/dp/B00W64H1Q4**
- **Is there audio for this book?** Yes, you can find the audiobook here: **https://adbl.co/2SwzzlA**

> *"Best resource I have found for explaining in terms I can understand about what my husband is experiencing and will be going through."*
>
> Kindle Customer

Reference List

American Academy of Orthopaedic Surgeons. (2012). Guidelines for preventing falls. Retrieved from http://orthoinfo.aaos.org/topic.cfm?topic=A00135.

Alzheimer's Association. (2012). Staying safe: Steps to take for a person with dementia. Retrieved from https://www.alz.org/national/documents/brochure_stayingsafe.pdf.

Alzheimer's Association. (2014). Retrieved from http://www.alz.org/.

Alzheimer's Compendium. (n.d.) Traveling with an Alzheimer's patient. Retrieved from http://www.alzcompend.info/?p=133.

Alzheimer's Foundation of America. (2014). Retrieved from http://www.alzfdn.org/index.htm.

Alzheimer's Hope. (2014). Wandering. Retrieved from http://www.alzheimershope.com/symptoms_strategies/wandering.php.

Alzheimer's Society. (2013). Mistreatment and abuse of people with dementia. Retrieved from http://www.alzheimers.org.uk/site/scripts/documents_info.php?documentID=422.

Alzheimer Society Canada. (2014). Holidays and special occasions. Retrieved from http://www.alzheimer.ca/en/Living-with-dementia/Staying-connected/Holidays-and-special-occasions.

Alzheimer Society of Manitoba. (2006). Fact sheet: Special occasions. Retrieved from http://www.alzheimer.mb.ca/wp-content/uploads/2013/09/Special-Occasions.pdf.

Barak, Y. & Aizenberg, D. (2002). Suicide amongst Alzheimer's disease patients: A 10-year survey. Dementia and Geriatric Cognitive Disorders, 14(2), 101-103.

Care Pathways. (2014). Home care agency checklist. Retrieved from http://www.carepathways.com/checklist-hc.cfm.

Fisher Center for Alzheimer's Research Foundation. (2014). Retrieved from http://www.alzinfo.org/.

Heerema, E. (2013). Elder abuse and Alzheimer's disease: Types, indicators, prevention and response to elder abuse. About Health. Retrieved from http://alzheimers.about.com/od/legalissues/a/Elder-Abuse-And-Alzheimers-Disease.htm.

Heerema, E. (2014). What to do when someone with dementia talks about suicide. About Health. Retrieved from http://alzheimers.about.com/od/behaviormanagement/a/What-To-Do-When-Someone-With-Dementia-Talks-About-Suicide.htm.

Mayo Clinic. (2013). Alzheimer's: When to stop driving. Retrieved from http://www.mayoclinic.org/healthy-living/caregivers/in-depth/alzheimers/art-20044924?pg=1.

National Institute on Aging. (2010). Home safety for people with Alzheimer's disease. Retrieved from http://www.nia.nih.gov/sites/default/files/home_safety_for_people_with_alzheimers_disease_2.pdf.

National Institute on Aging. (2011). Driving and dementia: Health professionals can play an important role. Retrieved from http://www.nia.nih.gov/alzheimers/features/driving-and-dementia-health-professionals-can-play-important-role.

Seyfried, L. S., Kales, H. C., Ignacio, R. V., Conwell, Y., & Valenstein, M. (2011). Predictors of suicide in patients with dementia. Alzheimer's & Dementia, 7(6), 567-573.

"Staying safe: Wandering and the Alzheimer's patient." (2012). Dementia Today. Retrieved from http://www.dementiatoday.com/staying-safe-wandering-and-the-alzheimers-patient/.

The Hartford Financial Services Group. (2010). At the crossroads: Family conversations about Alzheimer's disease, dementia & driving. Retrieved from http://hartfordauto.thehartford.com/UI/Downloads/Crossroads.pdf.

The Hartford Financial Services Group. (2010). The calm before the storm: Family conversations about disaster planning, caregiving, Alzheimer's disease, and dementia. Retrieved from http://hartfordauto.thehartford.com/UI/Downloads/CalmBeforeStor mBro.pdf.

Made in the USA
Monee, IL
18 May 2023